How to Use Essential Oils for Beginners

A Step-By-Step Guide to DIY Aromatherapy Recipes for Anxiety Relief, Sleep Remedies, All-Natural Cleaning Products, Skin Care, Pain Management, and More

The Fix-It Guy

Copyright © The Fix-It Guy

Table of Contents

Introduction

Welcome to the aromatic world of essential oils, where nature's fragrant wonders meet your everyday life! Have you ever dreamt of turning your home into a spa-like sanctuary, or effortlessly soothing away stress and anxiety with the power of scents? Well, dear reader, you've just stumbled upon the key to unlocking that fragrant treasure trove, "How to Use Essential Oils for Beginners: A Step-By-Step Guide to DIY Aromatherapy Recipes for Anxiety Relief, Sleep Remedies, All-Natural Cleaning Products, Skin Care, Pain Management, and More."

Now, I know what you might be thinking. Essential oils? DIY? Anxiety relief? Skincare? Is this some kind of magic potion cookbook? Well, not quite, but close enough! Think of it as your trusty guide to navigating the aromatic jungle of essential oils, where we'll arm you with the knowledge and recipes to turn your daily rituals into delightful, fragrant experiences.

Picture this: You, basking in the serene aroma of lavender as you bid farewell to the day's stress. Or perhaps, the subtle scent of eucalyptus wafting through your home, transforming cleaning chores into a spa-like cleanse for your living space. Intrigued? You should be! This book isn't just a guide; it's a journey into the world of scents that'll revolutionize the way you approach well-being.

But wait, there's more! Dive into the chapters, and you'll discover the secrets of crafting your sleep-inducing potions, banishing pain with the flick of an oil-drenched wrist, and even creating skincare miracles straight from your kitchen. It's a DIY extravaganza that promises not only to improve your well-being but also to turn you into the alchemist of your aromatic destiny.

So, buckle up, dear reader! Whether you're a seasoned aromatherapy enthusiast or a curious beginner, this book is your passport to a world where stress takes a back seat, sleep becomes a cherished friend, and your living space transforms into a fragrant haven. Let's embark on this aromatic adventure together, because who said self-care can't be as delightful as a bouquet of your favorite flowers? Get ready to unleash the magic of essential oils in your life!

Chapter 1

Understanding Essential Oils

What Are Essential Oils?

Hey there, Essential Explorer! Ready to dive into the fragrant wonderland of essential oils? Awesome, because we're about to unravel the mystery behind these tiny bottles of liquid magic. Imagine them as nature's little superheroes, each with a unique power to make your life a whole lot better. So, grab your cape (or cozy blanket, your call), and let's embark on this aromatic adventure!

What Are Essential Oils?

Alright, friend, let's keep it simple. Essential oils are like the soul of a plant, bottled up for your enjoyment. Think of them as the plant's way of saying, "Hey, here's my essence, my vibe, my secret sauce!" They're extracted from flowers, leaves, bark, and other plant parts. Now, don't worry about the sciencey stuff; just know that these oils are pure, potent, and packed with goodness.

Troubleshooting Tip: If you're wondering where to find these plant superheroes, your local health store or a trusted online retailer is your go-to sidekick.

Different Types of Essential Oils

You wouldn't wear flip-flops in a snowstorm, right? The same goes for essential oils, different oils, different jobs. Some oils are calming, others are energizing, and a few are multitasking geniuses. It's like assembling your Avengers team but for your senses.

Here's a quick cheat sheet:
- **Lavender:** The chill pill of essential oils.
- **Peppermint:** Your wake-up call in a bottle.
- **Tea Tree:** The superhero of clean and clear skin.

Troubleshooting Tip: Feeling overwhelmed with choices? Start with a few versatile oils and let your collection grow organically. No need to rush; it's not a race.

Extraction Methods and Quality Considerations

Alright, buckle up for a mini-ride into the making of these aromatic wonders. Extraction methods are like the secret handshake of the essential oil world. Steam distillation, cold-pressing – sounds like a spy movie, doesn't it? Each method brings out the best in different oils.

Quality Check Alert: Not all oils are created equal. Look for pure, undiluted oils without funky additives. It's like shopping for the ripest fruit – you want the good stuff.

Troubleshooting Tip: If you're unsure about an oil's quality, a quick sniff test can reveal a lot. Fresh, potent, and true to its plant roots? You're golden!

Now, that's the lowdown on what essential oils are and how to pick the cream of the crop. Next time, we'll get our hands dirty (in a good way) with some practical tips on getting started. Until then, keep sniffing and stay curious, Essential Explorer!

Different Types of Essential Oils

Welcome back, Essential Explorer! Now that you've got the scoop on what essential oils are, let's talk about the stars of the show – the oils themselves. It's like assembling your dream team, each with its unique superpowers. So, grab your cape (or cozy socks, your choice) as we explore the fantastic world of different essential oils!

1. Lavender: The Chill Pill

Ah, lavender, the zen master of essential oils. Need to unwind after a hectic day? Lavender's got your back. Its calming aroma is like a warm hug for your senses, helping you kick back and relax. Drop a few lavender droplets on your pillow, and sweet dreams are practically guaranteed.

2. Peppermint: Your Wake-Up Call in a Bottle

Feeling a bit sluggish? Meet peppermint, your instant energy boost. Just a whiff of this zesty oil can jolt your senses awake. It's like a splash of cold water but without the whole "water" part. Perfect for those mornings when coffee just won't cut it.

3. Tea Tree: The Superhero of Clear Skin

Meet your skincare sidekick, tea tree oil. This little powerhouse is known for its blemish-busting abilities.

Got a pesky pimple? Dab a bit of diluted tea tree oil, and watch it work its magic. Clear skin, here you come!

Troubleshooting Tip: Essential oils are potent, so a little goes a long way. Start with just a drop or two, and let the magic unfold gradually.

4. Eucalyptus: The Breath of Fresh Air

Got a stuffy nose or feeling a bit under the weather? Enter eucalyptus, the respiratory superhero. Its invigorating scent can make you feel like you're breathing in the crisp mountain air, even if you're stuck in the city. Ideal for creating your spa day at home.

5. Lemon: The Sunshine in a Bottle

Need a mood lift? Lemon essential oil is here to brighten your day. Its citrusy aroma is like a burst of sunshine, instantly lifting your spirits. Plus, it's a natural mood enhancer, the happy dance is optional but highly encouraged.

Troubleshooting Tip: Some oils can be photosensitive, so if you're planning a day in the sun, save your lemon-scented adventures for the evening.

Remember, Essential Explorer, these are just a few drops in the vast ocean of essential oils. Experiment, mix, and match to find your perfect blend.

Extraction Methods and Quality Considerations

Hey there, Essential Explorer! Now that you know your Lavenders from your Peppermints, let's dive into the backstage of essential oils, where the magic happens. It's like discovering the secret recipes behind your favorite dishes, only with more aromas and less cooking. So, put on your detective hat (or cozy beanie, your style) as we unravel the mystery of extraction methods and quality considerations in the essential oil world.

1. Extraction Methods: The Secret Handshake of Essential Oils

Imagine essential oils as superheroes, and extraction methods as their unique origin stories. Each method distinctly extracts the essence of plants, resulting in oils with different characteristics. Let's break it down:

Steam Distillation: This is like the granddaddy of extraction methods. Plants take a steamy sauna, and their essential oils are captured in the steam. When the steam cools, you're left with pure, concentrated goodness.

Cold-Pressing: Picture juicing, but for essential oils. Citrus oils, like Lemon and Orange, are often extracted this way. The peel gets a good squeeze, and the oil is collected, no heat is involved.

Troubleshooting Tip: Different oils, different methods. For delicate flowers, it's steam distillation; for robust peels, it's cold-pressing. Choose oils based on their extraction method mojo.

2. Quality Considerations: Sniffing Out the Good Stuff Now that you're an extraction method expert, let's talk about quality. Not all essential oils are created equal, and trust me, you want the good stuff. Here's how to separate the champs from the wannabes:

Purity Check: Your essential oil should be as pure as your grandma's intentions. Look for oils without additives, fillers, or funky business. The ingredient list should have just one item: the plant.

Sourcing Matters: Just like fine wine, the region matters. Where your oil comes from can influence its aroma and potency. Think of it as the difference between a local farmer's market and a supermarket – go for the farmers' market quality.

Troubleshooting Tip: If an essential oil promises to smell like cotton candy or last for days, it might be too good to be true. Stick to the authentic, true-to-nature scents.

3. Sniff Test: Your Nose Knows

Now, let's talk about the sniff test. A good-quality essential oil should smell fresh, potent, and true to its plant roots. If it's supposed to be lavender, make sure it doesn't smell like an artificial lavender-scented candle from the dollar store.

Troubleshooting Tip: If you're uncertain, compare the scent with a trusted source or take a whiff of the real plant. Your nose is your best detective.

So, there you have it, Essential Explorer, the backstage pass to the essential oil world. Next time, we'll roll up our sleeves and start concocting some DIY blends. Get ready to be the master mixologist of your aromatic journey! Until then, keep sniffing and stay curious.

Chapter 2

Essential Oils for Anxiety Relief

The Science Behind Aromatherapy for Anxiety

Hey there, Calm Crusader! Are you ready to tackle one of life's sneaky foes, anxiety? In this chapter, we're delving into the superhero realm of essential oils, specifically crafted to be your allies in the battle against stress and worry. Get your metaphorical cape on (or cozy hoodie, your call) because we're about to explore the science behind aromatherapy for anxiety.

The Science Behind Aromatherapy for Anxiety

Alright, buckle up for a mini-science lesson, but fear not, it's more like a chill chat over a cup of herbal tea. Aromatherapy isn't just about making things smell good; there's some serious science behind it, especially when it comes to combating anxiety.

Aromas and the Brain Dance:
When you inhale the aroma of essential oils, it's like sending a VIP invitation to your brain's olfactory system, the fancy term for your smell receptors. These receptors send signals straight to the brain's emotional center, known as the limbic system. Now, the limbic system is the mood maestro, responsible for emotions, memories, and, you guessed it, anxiety.

The Calming Crew, Lavender and Chamomile:
Meet the dynamic duo, lavender and chamomile. These oils are like the zen masters of the essential oil world. They contain compounds that interact with the brain's receptors, promoting relaxation and calming the nervous system. It's like a spa day for your brain!

Citrusy Sunshine, Bergamot and Sweet Orange:
Ever noticed how a whiff of citrus can instantly uplift your mood? Bergamot and sweet orange essential oils work their magic by boosting the levels of a neurotransmitter called serotonin. Higher serotonin equals a happier, less anxious you.

Troubleshooting Tip: Experiment with different oils to find your anxiety-busting sidekick. Your brain might groove to lavender's chill vibes, while your friend's brain might prefer the citrusy dance of bergamot. It's a personalized journey!

Top Essential Oils for Calming the Mind

Let's meet the anxiety-busting all-stars, shall we?

Lavender: The Crown Jewel of Calm

Known for its soothing properties, lavender is your go-to stress buster. Diffuse it, blend it, or even put a drop on your pillow for a tranquil night's sleep.

Chamomile: The Sleepytime Specialist

Chamomile isn't just for tea; its essential oil version is a bedtime game-changer. Inhale its gentle aroma to coax your mind into a state of serene relaxation.

Bergamot: The Citrusy Sunbeam

Need a mood boost? Bergamot is like sunshine in a bottle. Inhale its sweet, citrusy scent to lift your spirits and kick anxiety to the curb.

Sweet Orange: The Happy Dance Partner

If life's got you down, sweet orange is here to tango. Its vibrant aroma can energize your mind and chase away those anxious thoughts.

Troubleshooting Tip: Remember, the key is consistency. Incorporate these oils into your daily routine, whether through diffusing, topical application, or a calming bath. Your anxiety doesn't stand a chance against this aromatic dream team.

There you have it, Calm Crusader, the science-backed secrets of using essential oils to kick anxiety to the curb. In the next chapter, we'll get hands-on with some DIY anxiety relief blends. So, take a deep breath, inhale the calming aroma, and get ready for a journey to a stress-free state. Until then, keep calm and oil on!

DIY Anxiety Relief Blends

Hello, Anxiety Avenger! Now that we've unraveled the science behind aromatherapy for anxiety, it's time to get hands-on and concoct some superhero blends that'll have stress running for the hills. Consider this your DIY anxiety relief lab, where we'll mix, match, and blend our way to tranquility. Grab your mixing bowl (or a cup, no judgment) because we're about to become master mixologists of calm.

1. Lavender and Chamomile Dreamland Blend:

Ingredients:
- 5 drops of Lavender essential oil
- 3 drops Chamomile essential oil
- 2 tablespoons carrier oil (like sweet almond or jojoba)

Method:
1. Mix the essential oils and carrier oil in a small, dark-colored bottle.
2. Shake well to ensure a thorough blend.
3. Apply a few drops to your wrists, temples, or the back of your neck whenever anxiety comes knocking.

Why it Works:

Lavender and chamomile team up to create a calming symphony. Apply this blend before bedtime for a tranquil night's sleep or whenever you need a moment of serenity.

2. Citrusy Uplift Blend:

Ingredients:
- 4 drops of Bergamot essential oil
- 3 drops of Sweet Orange essential oil
- 1 drop of Peppermint essential oil
- 2 tablespoons carrier oil

Method:
1. Combine the essential oils and carrier oil in a bottle.
2. Give it a good shake to blend the oils.
3. Dab a small amount on your pulse points or inhale the refreshing aroma when anxiety strikes.

Why it Works:

Bergamot and sweet orange bring the sunshine, while a hint of peppermint adds a refreshing twist. This blend is perfect for boosting your mood and tackling stress head-on.

3. Calm and Ground Blend:

Ingredients:
- 4 drops of Frankincense essential oil
- 3 drops of Vetiver essential oil
- 2 drops of Lavender essential oil
- 2 tablespoons carrier oil

Method:
1. Mix the essential oils and carrier oil in a container.
2. Shake well to blend the oils thoroughly.
3. Apply to the bottoms of your feet or pulse points for a sense of grounding and calm.

Why it Works:
Frankincense and vetiver bring a sense of grounding, while lavender adds its calming touch. This blend is perfect for creating a serene atmosphere during moments of tension.

Troubleshooting Tip:
Remember, everyone's nose and preferences are different. Feel free to adjust the number of drops based on your scent preference, and always start with a lower concentration if you have sensitive skin.

There you have it, Anxiety Avenger, your arsenal of DIY anxiety relief blends. Experiment, find your favorites, and let the aromatic journey to tranquility begin. In the next chapter, we'll explore essential oils for a different kind of relaxation – the kind that leads to a restful night's sleep. Until then, keep blending and stay calm!

Chapter 3

Sleep Remedies with Essential Oils

Importance of Sleep for Well-being

Greetings, Restful Explorer! In this chapter, we're delving into the magical realm of essential oils designed to whisk you away to the land of dreams. Picture this as your passport to a restful night's sleep, where anxiety takes a back seat, and sweet dreams take the wheel. So, slip into your favorite pajamas (or sleep shorts, no judgment here), and let's explore the importance of sleep for your overall well-being.

Importance of Sleep for Well-being
Let's get real, we've all had those nights of tossing, turning, and counting imaginary sheep. But why does sleep matter so much, beyond the simple act of resting our eyes?

The Restoration Station:
Sleep is like a superhero for your body and mind, swooping in to restore and rejuvenate. During those peaceful slumber hours, your body works its magic,

repairing cells, boosting the immune system, and even consolidating memories. It's like a nightly spa treatment for your entire being.

Mood Manager:

Ever noticed how everything seems a bit more daunting after a sleepless night? That's not just your imagination – lack of sleep can mess with your mood, making stress feel more intense and joy a bit harder to find. A well-rested mind is a resilient mind, ready to tackle whatever comes your way.

Energy Refill:

Think of sleep as your body's way of recharging its batteries. It's not just about quantity; quality sleep ensures you wake up refreshed and ready to conquer the day. Forget about hitting the snooze button a dozen times, with proper sleep, you'll be up and at 'em with gusto.

Troubleshooting Tip:

Struggling with sleep? Before diving into essential oils, consider your sleep hygiene. Keep your sleep space cool, dark, and gadget-free, and establish a consistent bedtime routine. Now, let's add some aromatic flair to enhance your sleep sanctuary.

Essential Oils That Promote Relaxation

Welcome back, Restful Explorer! Now that we've laid the groundwork on the importance of a good night's sleep, let's dive into the aromatic world of essential oils that will transform your bedtime routine into a tranquil spa-like experience. Get ready to meet the dream team of essential oils that will whisk you away to the realm of relaxation.

1. Lavender: The Soothing Maestro

Ah, lavender, the rockstar of relaxation. This timeless classic is your go-to oil when you need to unwind. Its floral, sweet aroma has a magical ability to calm the nervous system, making it a perfect companion for bedtime bliss. Whether diffused, applied to your pillow, or added to a relaxing bath, lavender is a must-have in your relaxation toolkit.

2. Roman Chamomile: The Calming Companion

Chamomile isn't just for tea; its essential oil counterpart is a relaxation powerhouse. Known for its calming properties, Roman Chamomile helps soothe anxiety and ease the mind into a state of tranquility. A few drops in a diffuser or mixed with a carrier oil for a massage can work wonders before bedtime.

3. Bergamot: The Citrus Serenity

If you're looking for a citrusy twist to your relaxation routine, say hello to bergamot. Its bright, uplifting scent can help alleviate stress and create a positive atmosphere. Blend it with lavender for a delightful duo that promotes relaxation and a sense of well-being.

4. Ylang Ylang: The Floral Fantasy

Ylang-ylang is like a tropical vacation for your senses. Its rich, floral aroma is not only exotic but also has a sedative effect, promoting relaxation and balancing emotions. Add a few drops to your diffuser, and let the floral fantasy transport you to a serene state of mind.

Troubleshooting Tip:

Experiment with different oils or create your personalized blend by combining a couple of drops of your favorites. Everyone's relaxation cocktail is unique, so don't be afraid to mix and match until you find the perfect harmony for your senses.

Creating a Relaxation Ritual:

Now that you've met the essential oil all-stars, let's turn this into a bedtime ritual:

1. Diffuser Delight: Add a few drops of your chosen essential oil to a diffuser in your bedroom. Let the gentle mist create a soothing ambiance.

2. Massage Magic: Mix a couple of drops of your preferred oil with a carrier oil and give yourself a relaxing foot or neck massage before bedtime.

3. Bedtime Bath Bliss: Add a few drops of your chosen oils to your evening bath. Picture it as a fragrant soak into dreamland.

4. Pillow Perfume: Place a drop or two of essential oil on your pillow or a cotton ball near your bed for a subtle, calming scent.

There you have it, Restful Explorer, the aromatic companions that will guide you to the land of relaxation. In the next chapter, we'll take these oils and blend them into DIY sleep-inducing potions. Get ready for a bedtime routine that'll have you drifting off to dreamland in no time. Until then, relax, breathe, and enjoy the calming embrace of essential oils.

Creating Your Own Sleep-Inducing Blends

Ahoy, Dreamweaver! Now that you've met the essential oil rockstars of relaxation, it's time to play mad scientist and concoct your very own sleep-inducing potions. Imagine this as a DIY adventure, where you blend, mix, and create the perfect aromatic symphony for your bedtime routine. So, gather your essential oils, put on your mixing hat (or just use your regular hat, it's your show), and let's dive into the art of creating personalized sleep-inducing blends.

1. Lavender-Chamomile Slumber Elixir:

Ingredients:
- 4 drops of Lavender essential oil
- 3 drops Roman Chamomile essential oil
- 2 drops Ylang Ylang essential oil
- 2 tablespoons carrier oil (like jojoba or almond)

Method:
1. In a dark-colored bottle, combine the essential oils with the carrier oil.
2. Give it a good shake to ensure the oils are thoroughly mixed.
3. Apply a small amount to your wrists, temples, or the soles of your feet before bedtime.

Why it Works:
Lavender and chamomile bring their relaxation magic, while ylang-ylang adds a touch of floral sweetness. This blend is a bedtime serenade for your senses.

2. Citrus Bliss Dream Mist:

Ingredients:
- 3 drops of Bergamot essential oil
- 3 drops of Sweet Orange essential oil
- 2 drops Frankincense essential oil
- 1 tablespoon witch hazel or distilled water

Method:
1. In a spray bottle, combine the essential oils with witch hazel or distilled water.
2. Shake well before misting your bedroom, pillows, or sleep space.

Why it Works:
Bergamot and sweet orange bring a burst of citrusy joy, while frankincense adds a grounding element. Spritz this mist for a refreshing pre-sleep atmosphere.

3. Tranquil Twilight Roller Blend:

Ingredients:
- 4 drops of Lavender essential oil

- 3 drops of Vetiver essential oil
- 2 drops Cedarwood essential oil
- 2 tablespoons fractionated coconut oil

Method:

1. Mix the essential oils with fractionated coconut oil in a roller bottle.

2. Roll onto your wrists, neck, or pulse points before bedtime.

Why it Works:

Lavender provides a calming base, vetiver adds grounding vibes, and cedarwood contributes a woodsy touch. Roll on and let the tranquility unfold.

Troubleshooting Tip:

Feel free to tweak the number of drops based on your scent preferences. If you find a blend too potent, dilute it with a bit more carrier oil. The goal is to create a scent that feels just right for you.

There you have it, Dreamweaver, your personalized sleep-inducing blends. Experiment, explore, and let your senses guide you to the perfect nighttime elixir. In the next chapter, we'll explore more practical tips for incorporating these blends into your nightly routine. Sweet dreams and happy blending!

Chapter 4

All-Natural Cleaning Products

Ditching Harmful Chemicals in Cleaning

Hey there, In this chapter, we're taking a detour from bedtime bliss and stepping into the world of sparkling countertops and fresh-scented homes. Get ready to revolutionize your cleaning routine as we explore the wonders of all-natural cleaning products. Say goodbye to harsh chemicals, and let's usher in a new era of cleanliness that's safe for you, your family, and the planet.

Ditching Harmful Chemicals in Cleaning

Let's face it, the cleaning aisle at the store can be overwhelming. Endless bottles filled with promises of cleanliness, but at what cost? Many commercial cleaning products contain a cocktail of harsh chemicals that might get the job done but can leave behind a trail of environmental and health concerns.

The Trouble with Traditional Cleaners:

Chemical-laden cleaners can release harmful fumes into the air, irritate the skin, and contribute to indoor air pollution. Plus, let's not forget the environmental impact of those plastic bottles piling up in landfills.

The Allure of All-Natural Cleaning:

Enter the superheroes of the cleaning world, all-natural cleaning products. These DIY wonders not only get the job done but do so without the negative side effects. You'll be amazed at how simple ingredients like vinegar, baking soda, and essential oils can tackle grime and leave your home smelling like a fragrant garden.

Troubleshooting Tip:

If you're worried about the efficacy of natural cleaners, fear not! The power of ingredients like vinegar and baking soda is backed by generations of homemakers who knew a thing or two about keeping homes spick and span.

Essential Oils for All-Natural Cleaning

Before we dive into specific recipes, let's talk about the cleaning superheroes, essential oils. These potent extracts aren't just for relaxation; they're also fantastic for cutting through grease, eliminating odors, and adding a fresh scent to your cleaning routine. Here are a few essential oils to keep in your green cleaning arsenal:

1. Lemon: A natural degreaser and antiseptic, lemon oil leaves surfaces sparkling clean and smelling fresh.

2. Tea Tree: With its antibacterial and antifungal properties, tea tree oil is perfect for tackling mold and mildew.

3. Peppermint: Known for its invigorating scent, peppermint oil is great for banishing musty odors and keeping pests at bay.

4. Lavender: Beyond its calming properties, lavender oil has antibacterial and antiviral qualities, making it a versatile addition to your cleaners.

DIY All-Purpose Cleaner:

Ingredients:
- 1 cup distilled white vinegar
- 1 cup water
- 20 drops of tea tree essential oil
- 10 drops of lavender essential oil

Method:

1. Combine all ingredients in a spray bottle.
2. Shake well before each use.
3. Spray onto surfaces and wipe with a clean cloth.

Why it Works:

Vinegar cuts through grease and grime, while tea tree and lavender oils add antibacterial and antiviral power, leaving your surfaces clean and refreshed.

Baking Soda Scrub:

Ingredients:

- ½ cup baking soda
- Enough water to form a paste
- 10 drops of lemon essential oil

Method:

1. Mix baking soda and water to form a paste.
2. Add lemon essential oil and stir well.
3. Apply the paste to surfaces, scrub, and rinse.

Why it Works:

Baking soda acts as a gentle abrasive, while lemon oil adds a refreshing scent and boosts the cleaning power.

Simple DIY Cleaning Recipes

Hello there, Green Clean Enthusiast! Now that we've discussed the why, let's jump into the how. In this section, we'll explore simple and effective DIY cleaning recipes that harness the power of natural ingredients and essential oils. Get ready to transform your cleaning routine into a fragrant and eco-friendly experience.

1. Citrus Infused Vinegar Cleaner:

Ingredients:
- Citrus peels (lemons, oranges, or grapefruits)
- Distilled white vinegar
- A glass jar with a lid

Method:
1. Fill the glass jar with citrus peels.
2. Pour distilled white vinegar over the peels until they are completely submerged.
3. Seal the jar and let it sit in a cool, dark place for at least two weeks.
4. Strain the vinegar into a spray bottle and dilute with equal parts water.

How to Use:
Spray on surfaces and wipe with a clean cloth. The citrus-infused vinegar acts as a powerful degreaser and leaves behind a fresh scent.

2. *Grease-Busting Lemon Dishwasher Tabs:*

Ingredients:
- 1 cup washing soda
- 1 cup baking soda
- 1 cup citric acid
- ½ cup coarse salt
- 30 drops of lemon essential oil
- Water (as needed)

Method:
1. In a large bowl, mix washing soda, baking soda, citric acid, and salt.
2. Add lemon essential oil and stir well.
3. Slowly add water, a little at a time, until the mixture holds together.
4. Pack the mixture into silicone molds and let them dry for 24 hours.

How to Use:
Place one tab in your dishwasher dispenser for a burst of citrusy freshness and grease-fighting power.

3. *Minty-Fresh All-Purpose Spray:*

Ingredients:
- 1 cup distilled white vinegar
- 1 cup water
- 20 drops of peppermint essential oil

Method:
1. Mix vinegar and water in a spray bottle.
2. Add peppermint essential oil and shake well.

How to Use:

Spray on countertops, surfaces, and even bathroom fixtures. The peppermint oil not only cleans but leaves a delightful, invigorating scent.

4. *Sparkling Glass and Mirror Cleaner:*

Ingredients:
- 1 cup distilled white vinegar
- 1 cup water
- 10 drops of lemon essential oil

Method:
1. Combine vinegar and water in a spray bottle.
2. Add lemon essential oil and shake well.

How to Use:
Spray on glass surfaces and mirrors, then wipe with a lint-free cloth for a streak-free shine and a burst of citrus freshness.

Troubleshooting Tip:
Feel free to adjust the number of essential oil drops based on your scent preferences. You can also experiment with different oils to create a signature scent for your cleaning arsenal.

There you have it, Green Clean Enthusiast – simple yet powerful DIY cleaning recipes to elevate your cleaning routine. In the next chapter, we'll explore tips and tricks for maintaining a clean and naturally fresh home. Happy cleaning!

Chapter 5

Essential Oils for Skin Care

Nourishing Your Skin Naturally

Greetings, Skin Care Enthusiast! In this chapter, we're diving into the world of radiant, healthy skin with the help of essential oils. Say goodbye to complicated skincare routines filled with mysterious ingredients, and welcome the simplicity of natural nourishment. Get ready to pamper your skin with the goodness of essential oils and unlock the secrets to a glowing complexion.

The Beauty of Natural Skin Care
Our skin is a remarkable organ, and treating it with care goes beyond mere aesthetics. Natural skincare is like a feast for your skin, providing it with the nutrients it needs to shine. Essential oils, derived from plants, bring a bouquet of benefits, from moisturizing to soothing and even combating blemishes.

The Essence of Essential Oils:
Essential oils are concentrated plant extracts, each with its unique set of properties. From lavender's calming

touch to tea tree's blemish-busting prowess, these oils can be your skin's best friend. By incorporating them into your skincare routine, you're giving your skin a taste of nature's goodness.

Essential Oils for Common Skin Concerns

1. Lavender for Calming and Soothing:

Benefits: Lavender oil is a multitasking marvel, known for its soothing properties. It can help reduce redness and irritation, and promote overall skin balance.

How to Use: Mix a few drops with a carrier oil for a gentle facial massage or add a drop to your daily moisturizer.

2. Tea Tree for Blemish Control:

Benefits: Tea tree oil is a natural antiseptic, making it excellent for managing acne and blemishes. It helps cleanse the skin and prevent breakouts.

How to Use: Apply a drop of tea tree oil to a cotton swab and dab it on affected areas. Remember to dilute with a carrier oil if applying directly to the skin.

3. Frankincense for Anti-Aging:

Benefits: Frankincense is like a time-traveling elixir, renowned for its anti-aging properties. It helps reduce the appearance of fine lines and promotes skin elasticity.

How to Use: Mix a few drops with your favorite facial oil or moisturizer and apply before bedtime.

4. Rosehip for Hydration and Radiance:

Benefits: Rosehip oil is a hydration hero, packed with vitamins and antioxidants. It helps moisturize the skin, improve texture, and enhance radiance.

How to Use: Apply a few drops directly to the skin or mix with your favorite lotion for an extra boost of hydration.

Troubleshooting Tip:

Always perform a patch test before applying essential oils directly to your skin, especially if you have sensitive skin or are trying a new oil. It's better to be safe than sorry!

DIY Essential Oil Face Serum:

Ingredients:
- 1 tablespoon jojoba oil
- 1 tablespoon rosehip oil
- 4 drops of lavender essential oil
- 3 drops frankincense essential oil

Method:

1. In a dark glass bottle, combine jojoba and rosehip oils.
2. Add the essential oils and shake well to mix.
3. Apply a few drops to your face and neck after cleansing.

Why it Works:
Jojoba and rosehip oils provide a nourishing base, while lavender and frankincense contribute their skincare superpowers. This DIY serum is a treat for your skin, leaving it hydrated, radiant, and balanced.

There you have it, Skin Care Enthusiast – the gateway to naturally nourished and radiant skin. In the next chapter, we'll explore the world of essential oils for pain management, so get ready to soothe those aches and pains naturally. Until then, enjoy the glow!

Best Essential Oils for Different Skin Types

Hello, Radiant Complexion Seeker! One size does not fit all when it comes to skincare, and that's where essential oils swoop in as your personalized skin superheroes. In this section, we'll explore the best essential oils tailored to different skin types, ensuring that your skincare routine is as unique as you are. Get ready to unveil the secret to a skin-loving regimen that suits your individual needs.

1. For Dry Skin:

Argan Oil:
Benefits: Argan oil is a hydration powerhouse, rich in essential fatty acids and vitamin E. It nourishes dry skin, restoring moisture and promoting a supple complexion.

Rose Otto:
Benefits: Rose Otto is like a floral hug for your skin. It helps soothe dryness, reduces redness, and provides a luxurious aroma. A true treat for dehydrated skin.

2. For Oily/Acne-Prone Skin:

Tea Tree:

Benefits: Tea tree oil is a blemish-busting champion. Its natural antibacterial properties help control acne and breakouts, keeping your skin clear and refreshed.

Geranium:

Benefits: Geranium oil balances oil production, making it an excellent choice for oily skin. It also has a pleasant floral scent that uplifts your senses.

3. For Sensitive Skin:

Chamomile:

Benefits: Chamomile is a gentle giant, known for its anti-inflammatory and soothing properties. It helps calm sensitive skin, making it a go-to for those prone to redness or irritation.

Calendula:

Benefits: Calendula oil is a calming companion for sensitive skin. It supports skin healing and reduces inflammation, making it perfect for delicate complexions.

4. For Combination Skin:

Lavender:

Benefits: Lavender is a versatile oil that suits most skin types, including combination skin. It helps balance oil production, soothes irritations, and promotes an even skin tone.

Frankincense:
Benefits: Frankincense is a harmonizing oil that works well for combination skin. It helps even out the skin's texture, reduces the appearance of pores, and supports overall skin health.

5. For Mature/Aging Skin:

Rosehip Seed:
Benefits: Rosehip seed oil is a potent anti-aging elixir. Packed with vitamins A and C, it helps diminish fine lines, improve skin tone, and restore youthful radiance.

Carrot Seed:
Benefits: Carrot seed oil is rich in antioxidants, promoting skin renewal and addressing signs of aging. It's a rejuvenating oil that supports mature skin beautifully.

Troubleshooting Tip:
Feel free to experiment with different oils to find the perfect match for your skin. You can also create your custom blends by combining oils that cater to your specific needs.

Chapter 6

Pain Management with Essential Oils

Understanding Pain and Aromatherapy

Hello, Pain Warrior! In this chapter, we're stepping into the realm of soothing scents and natural relief. Whether it's a persistent ache or a fleeting pain, essential oils have the potential to be your allies in the battle against discomfort. So, let's unravel the connection between pain and aromatherapy, and discover how these aromatic wonders can offer relief for various types of discomfort.

Understanding Pain:
Pain is like an unwelcome guest that can manifest in various forms, from headaches and muscle soreness to chronic conditions like arthritis. Understanding the nature of your pain is the first step in finding effective relief.

Types of Pain:
1. Muscle Pain: Caused by tension, strain, or overuse of muscles.

2. Joint Pain: Often associated with conditions like arthritis or injury.

3. Headache/Migraine: A common discomfort that can range from mild to severe.

4. Nerve Pain: Resulting from nerve damage or conditions like sciatica.

Aromatherapy and Pain Relief:
Aromatherapy, the art of using essential oils to enhance well-being, has been used for centuries to alleviate various ailments, including pain. The aromatic compounds in essential oils interact with the olfactory system, sending signals to the brain that can influence mood, emotions, and even pain perception.

Essential Oils for Pain Relief:
1. Peppermint: Known for its cooling sensation, peppermint oil can help relieve headaches and muscle tension.

2. Eucalyptus: With its anti-inflammatory properties, eucalyptus oil is great for soothing muscle and joint pain.

3. Lavender: Famous for its calming effects, lavender oil can help reduce stress-related pain and headaches.

4. Ginger: A warming oil, ginger can be beneficial for muscle and joint pain, especially in conditions like arthritis.

5. Chamomile: With anti-inflammatory and relaxing properties, chamomile oil is excellent for calming nerve pain and muscle discomfort.

DIY Pain-Relief Blends:

1. Soothing Muscle Massage Oil:

Ingredients:
- 2 tablespoons carrier oil (like sweet almond or jojoba)
- 5 drops peppermint essential oil
- 3 drops eucalyptus essential oil

Method:
1. Mix the essential oils with the carrier oil.
2. Massage the blend onto sore muscles for relief.

2. Headache Relief Roll-On:

Ingredients:
- 1 tablespoon fractionated coconut oil
- 3 drops of lavender essential oil
- 2 drops peppermint essential oil

Method:
1. Mix the essential oils with fractionated coconut oil.
2. Apply the roll-on to your temples and massage gently.

Troubleshooting Tip:
Always perform a patch test before applying essential oils directly to your skin. If you have a specific medical condition or are pregnant, consult with a healthcare professional before using essential oils for pain management.

There you have it, Pain Warrior, a glimpse into the world of pain management with essential oils. In the next chapter, we'll explore how these aromatic wonders can enhance your overall well-being, from boosting mood to promoting relaxation. Until then, may your pain be fleeting, and your relief aromatic!

Essential Oils for Pain Relief

Greetings, Relief Seeker! Essential oils, the aromatic champions of nature, hold incredible potential in providing comfort and alleviating various types of pain. In this section, we'll explore the specific essential oils renowned for their pain-relieving properties, offering you a natural pathway to relief. Get ready to harness the power of these botanical wonders for a soothing and aromatic journey.

1. Peppermint Oil:

Benefits:
Cooling Sensation: Peppermint oil contains menthol, providing a cooling sensation that can soothe headaches and muscle tension.
Anti-Inflammatory: Its anti-inflammatory properties make it effective for reducing pain associated with sore muscles and joints.

How to Use:
- Dilute with a carrier oil and massage onto the affected area.
- Inhale the aroma through steam inhalation or diffusing.

2. Eucalyptus Oil:

Benefits:
Anti-Inflammatory and Analgesic: Eucalyptus oil's anti-inflammatory and analgesic properties can help ease muscle and joint pain.
Respiratory Relief: It's also beneficial for respiratory-related discomfort, providing relief to conditions like sinus congestion.

How to Use:
- Dilute and apply topically to the affected area.
- Inhale the vapors through steam inhalation or diffusing.

3. Lavender Oil:

Benefits:
Calming and Relaxing: Lavender oil's calming effects make it effective for reducing stress-related pain and tension headaches.
Anti-Inflammatory: It has mild anti-inflammatory properties, contributing to pain relief.

How to Use:
- Dilute with a carrier oil for a relaxing massage.
- Add a few drops to a warm bath for overall relaxation.

4. *Ginger Oil:*

Benefits:
Warming Sensation: Ginger oil provides a warming sensation, making it beneficial for soothing muscle and joint pain.
Anti-Inflammatory: It has anti-inflammatory properties that can assist in relieving pain associated with arthritis.

How to Use:
- Dilute with a carrier oil and massage onto the affected area.
- Inhale the aroma through steam inhalation or diffusing.

5. *Chamomile Oil:*

Benefits:
Anti-Inflammatory and Calming: Chamomile oil's anti-inflammatory properties make it useful for calming nerve pain and reducing inflammation.
Muscle Relaxant: It acts as a gentle muscle relaxant, aiding in relieving tension.

How to Use:
- Dilute with a carrier oil for a calming massage.
- Add a few drops to a warm compress for targeted relief.

Troubleshooting Tip:
Experiment with single oils or create your blends based on your preferences. Everyone's response to essential oils can vary, so finding what works best for you is key.

There you have it, Relief Seeker, a guide to essential oils for pain relief. In the next chapter, we'll explore how these aromatic wonders can elevate your mood and enhance emotional well-being. Until then, may your pain be eased, and your senses delighted!

Crafting Pain-Relieving Blends

Hello, Blend Artisan! Now that you're familiar with the individual superheroes of pain relief, let's dive into the art of crafting your pain-relieving blends. Picture this as your aromatic apothecary, where you become the maestro, blending essential oils to create symphonies of relief for your unique needs. So, gather your oils, roll up your sleeves (figuratively, of course), and let the blending begin!

1. Soothing Muscle Melt Blend:

Ingredients:
- 3 drops Peppermint oil
- 2 drops Eucalyptus oil
- 2 drops Lavender oil
- 2 tablespoons carrier oil (like jojoba or almond)

Method:
1. In a dark-colored bottle, combine the essential oils with the carrier oil.
2. Mix well by rolling the bottle between your palms.
3. Apply the blend to sore muscles and gently massage for relief.

Why it Works:
Peppermint's cooling sensation, combined with the anti-inflammatory properties of eucalyptus and the calming touch of lavender, creates a trifecta of relief for achy muscles.

2. Headache Helper Roller Blend:

Ingredients:
- 2 drops Peppermint oil
- 2 drops Lavender oil
- 1 drop Eucalyptus oil
- 1 drop Chamomile oil
- 1 tablespoon fractionated coconut oil

Method:
1. In a roller bottle, combine the essential oils with fractionated coconut oil.
2. Roll onto your temples and gently massage for headache relief.

Why it Works:
Peppermint and lavender team up to ease tension, while eucalyptus provides a refreshing kick. Chamomile adds a calming touch for overall headache relief.

3. *Joint Soother Salve:*

Ingredients:
- 3 drops Ginger oil
- 2 drops Eucalyptus oil
- 2 drops Lavender oil
- 2 tablespoons shea butter or coconut oil

Method:
1. In a small container, melt the shea butter or coconut oil.
2. Add the essential oils and mix well.
3. Allow the mixture to solidify before applying to joints for relief.

Why it Works:
Ginger's warming sensation, combined with the anti-inflammatory properties of eucalyptus and the soothing touch of lavender, creates a balm for achy joints.

4. *Calm and Comfort Compress:*

Ingredients:
- 2 drops Chamomile oil
- 2 drops Lavender oil
- 1 drop of Peppermint oil
- Warm water

- Cotton cloth

Method:
1. Fill a bowl with warm water and add the essential oils.
2. Stir the water to disperse the oils.
3. Soak a cotton cloth in the mixture, wring out excess water, and place it on the affected area.

Why it Works:
Chamomile and lavender bring their calming properties, while peppermint adds a touch of coolness for a soothing compress.

Troubleshooting Tip:
Feel free to adjust the number of drops based on your preferences. If you find a blend too potent, dilute it further with carrier oil.

There you have it, Blend Artisan, your guide to crafting pain-relieving blends. In the next chapter, we'll explore how essential oils can be your allies in promoting emotional well-being. Until then, happy blending, and may your blends bring you the relief you seek!

Chapter 7

Other Practical Uses of Essential Oils

Aromatherapy for Focus and Concentration

Greetings, Seeker of Clarity! In this chapter, we're shifting gears to explore how essential oils can be your allies in the pursuit of enhanced focus and concentration. Whether you're navigating a demanding workday or aiming to boost your study sessions, aromatherapy has the power to elevate your mental clarity and sharpen your focus. Let's dive into the aromatic world of productivity and cognitive enhancement.

The Aroma-Mind Connection:
The connection between scent and the mind is a fascinating dance. Certain aromas can stimulate the brain, influencing mood, alertness, and cognitive function. Harnessing this power can be a game-changer in creating an environment that supports focus and concentration.

Essential Oils for Focus and Concentration:

1. Rosemary:

Benefits: Rosemary is like a herbal boost for the brain. It's known to improve memory, alertness, and overall cognitive performance.

2. Peppermint:

Benefits: Peppermint's invigorating scent can help stimulate the mind, enhance focus, and reduce mental fatigue.

3. Lemon:

Benefits: The bright and citrusy aroma of lemon oil is excellent for promoting a clear mind and boosting concentration.

4. Eucalyptus:

Benefits: Eucalyptus oil can invigorate the senses, helping to clear mental fog and improve concentration.

DIY Focus-Enhancing Diffuser Blend:

Ingredients:
- 3 drops Rosemary oil
- 2 drops Peppermint oil
- 2 drops Lemon oil
- 1 drop of Eucalyptus oil

Method:

1. Add the essential oils to your diffuser.

2. Turn on the diffuser in your workspace or study area.

Why it Works:

Rosemary brings mental clarity, peppermint adds an invigorating kick, lemon provides a refreshing boost, and eucalyptus clears the mental path. Together, they create a focused and energizing atmosphere.

Roll-On Energizing Blend:

Ingredients:

- 1 tablespoon carrier oil (such as jojoba or almond)
- 3 drops Rosemary oil
- 2 drops Peppermint oil
- 1 drop Lemon oil

Method:

1. Mix the essential oils with the carrier oil in a roller bottle.

2. Apply the blend to your pulse points, such as wrists and temples.

Why it Works:
This roll-on blend is a portable focus booster. The combination of rosemary, peppermint, and lemon keeps your mind sharp and alert throughout the day.

Troubleshooting Tip:
Experiment with the ratio of oils to find a blend that resonates with your preferences. Adjust the number of drops based on the strength you desire.

There you have it, Seeker of Clarity – a guide to using essential oils for enhanced focus and concentration. In the next chapter, we'll explore how these aromatic wonders can contribute to a calming and stress-free environment. Until then, may your mind be sharp, and your focus unwavering!

Essential Oils in Massage and Relaxation Techniques

Hello, Relaxation Enthusiast! In this chapter, we'll embark on a journey into the world of soothing massages and relaxation techniques enhanced by the magic of essential oils. Picture a serene space, calming scents, and the gentle touch of massage, the perfect recipe for unwinding and melting away stress. Let's explore how essential oils can elevate your relaxation experience to new heights.

The Harmony of Aromatherapy and Massage:
The combination of aromatherapy and massage is like a symphony for the senses. As skilled hands work their magic, the aromatic dance of essential oils enhances the experience, promoting relaxation, and creating a sense of well-being.

Essential Oils for Relaxation:

1. Lavender:
Benefits: Lavender is the superstar of relaxation. Its calming properties help reduce stress, promote tranquility, and contribute to a restful atmosphere.

2. Chamomile:
Benefits: Chamomile oil is a gentle sedative, making it ideal for promoting relaxation and easing tension.

3. Ylang Ylang:
Benefits: Ylang-ylang is known for its floral and exotic aroma, promoting a sense of calm and lifting the mood.

4. Frankincense:
Benefits: Frankincense has grounding properties that help create a serene environment, perfect for relaxation.

DIY Relaxing Massage Oil:

Ingredients:
- 2 tablespoons carrier oil (such as sweet almond or jojoba)
- 5 drops of Lavender oil
- 3 drops Chamomile oil
- 2 drops Ylang Ylang oil

Method:
1. Mix the essential oils with the carrier oil in a dark glass bottle.
2. Warm the oil before use by placing the bottle in a bowl of warm water.
3. Massage onto the body using gentle, rhythmic strokes.

Why it Works:
Lavender brings a sense of calm, chamomile adds a gentle touch, and ylang-ylang contributes to a blissful atmosphere, creating the perfect blend for relaxation.

Aromatherapy Diffusion during Massage:

Ingredients:
- Aromatherapy diffuser
- 3 drops Lavender oil
- 2 drops Frankincense oil

Method:
1. Add the essential oils to your aromatherapy diffuser.
2. Begin the massage in a room filled with the calming aroma.

Why it Works:
The diffusion of lavender and frankincense creates a tranquil environment, enhancing the overall relaxation experience.

Troubleshooting Tip:
Communicate with your massage therapist about your preferences and any sensitivities you may have to specific oils.

There you have it, Relaxation Enthusiast – a guide to incorporating essential oils into massage and relaxation techniques. In the next chapter, we'll explore how these aromatic wonders can contribute to a restful night's sleep. Until then, may your massages be soothing, and your relaxation profound!

Using Essential Oils in Daily Life

Greetings, Everyday Alchemist! In this chapter, we'll unravel the secrets of seamlessly integrating essential oils into your daily routine. From waking up in the morning to winding down at night, these aromatic wonders can be your companions, enhancing various aspects of your life. Get ready to discover the art of incorporating essential oils into the tapestry of your day.

Morning Energizer:
Start your day with a burst of energy and positivity.

Citrus Wake-Up Blend:

Ingredients:
- 3 drops Orange oil
- 2 drops Grapefruit oil
- 1 drop of Peppermint oil

Method:
1. Add the essential oils to your diffuser.
2. Inhale the invigorating aroma to kickstart your day.

Midday Refresh:
Combat the midday slump and stay focused.

Minty Focus Roller:

Ingredients:
- 1 tablespoon fractionated coconut oil
- 3 drops Peppermint oil
- 2 drops Rosemary oil

Method:
1. Mix the essential oils with the carrier oil in a roller bottle.
2. Apply to pulse points for a quick pick-me-up.

Stress-Free Afternoon:
Ease stress and promote a sense of calm.

Desk Relaxation Diffusion:

Ingredients:
- Aromatherapy diffuser
- 3 drops Lavender oil
- 2 drops Bergamot oil

Method:
1. Place the diffuser on your desk.
2. Enjoy the soothing aroma while working.

Evening Unwind:
The transition from the hustle to relaxation mode.

Cozy Evening Blend:

Ingredients:
- 3 drops Lavender oil
- 2 drops Cedarwood oil
- 1 drop of Frankincense oil

Method:
1. Add the essential oils to your bedside diffuser.
2. Let the calming scents guide you into a peaceful evening.

Nighttime Ritual:
Prepare for a restful night's sleep.

Sleepytime Linen Spray:

Ingredients:
- 2 ounces distilled water
- 1 tablespoon witch hazel
- 5 drops Chamomile oil
- 3 drops Lavender oil

Method:
1. Mix the essential oils with water and witch hazel in a spray bottle.
2. Spritz on your pillow and bedding before sleep.

On-the-Go Support:
Bring the benefits of essential oils wherever you go.

Stress-Relief Inhaler:

Ingredients:
- Blank inhaler tube
- 5 drops Bergamot oil
- 3 drops Frankincense oil

Method:
1. Add the essential oils to the inhaler tube.
2. Inhale deeply whenever you need a moment of calm.

Troubleshooting Tip:
Remember to perform patch tests and be mindful of any sensitivities. Adjust the number of drops based on your preferences.

There you have it, Everyday Alchemist, a guide to incorporating essential oils into your daily life. In the next chapter, we'll explore advanced techniques for those ready to delve deeper into the world of aromatherapy.

Chapter 8

Safety Tips and Precautions

Dilution Guidelines

Hello, Safety Navigator! In this crucial chapter, we'll delve into the guidelines and precautions that ensure your journey into the world of essential oils is not only enjoyable but also safe. Essential oils are potent and concentrated, and understanding how to use them responsibly is paramount. Let's equip you with the knowledge to navigate the aromatic realm safely.

Dilution Guidelines:
Essential oils are powerful, and proper dilution is key to ensuring their safe application.

General Dilution Guidelines:

For Adults:
- 1–2% dilution for regular use (1–2 drops per teaspoon of carrier oil).
- 2.5–5% dilution for localized application (2–5 drops per teaspoon of carrier oil).

For Children (ages 2–12):

- 0.5–1% dilution for regular use (1–2 drops per 2 teaspoons of carrier oil).
- 1–2.5% dilution for localized application (1–2 drops per teaspoon of carrier oil).

For Infants (ages 0–2):

- 0.1–0.25% dilution for regular use (1 drop per 4 teaspoons of carrier oil).
- 0.25–0.5% dilution for localized application (1 drop per 2 teaspoons of carrier oil).

Allergies and Sensitivities with Safe Practices for Using Essential Oils

While essential oils are natural, allergic reactions or sensitivities can still occur.

Patch Testing:
- Always perform a patch test before applying an essential oil to a larger area.
- Apply a small diluted amount of the oil on the inner forearm and wait for 24–48 hours to check for any adverse reactions.

Common Allergens:
- Be aware of potential allergens like nuts (as carrier oils), citrus oils, and specific floral oils.
- If you have known allergies, consult with a healthcare professional before using new essential oils.

Safe Practices for Using Essential Oils:

Storage:
- Store essential oils in dark glass bottles in a cool, dry place away from direct sunlight.
- Keep oils out of reach of children and pets.

Application:

- Dilute essential oils before applying them to the skin.
- Use a carrier oil like sweet almond, jojoba, or coconut oil for dilution.

Ingestion:

- Exercise caution when ingesting essential oils. Not all oils are safe for internal use.
- Consult with a qualified aromatherapist or healthcare professional before ingesting essential oils.

Phototoxic Oils:

- Some citrus oils, like bergamot, can cause skin sensitivity in the sun.
- Avoid sun exposure on areas where phototoxic oils have been applied.

Pregnancy and Medical Conditions:

Consult with a healthcare professional before using essential oils during pregnancy or if you have underlying health conditions.

Emergency Measures:

In Case of Accidental Ingestion:
- Contact a poison control center immediately.
- Do not induce vomiting unless advised by medical professionals.

For Eye Contact:
- Rinse eyes with a carrier oil, not water, to dilute the oil.
- Seek medical attention if irritation persists.

Troubleshooting Tip:
When in doubt, start with a lower dilution and increase gradually. Listen to your body, and if you experience any adverse reactions, discontinue use.

There you have it, Safety Navigator – a comprehensive guide to safety tips and precautions in the world of essential oils. In the next chapter, we'll explore advanced techniques for those ready to deepen their understanding and practice of aromatherapy. Until then, may your aromatic journey be both enjoyable and safe!

Guidelines and precautions that ensure your journey into the world of essential oils is not only enjoyable but also safe.

Conclusion

As we bid adieu to this aromatic expedition, it's time to reflect on the incredible odyssey we've shared in "How to Use Essential Oils for Beginners." From unraveling the mysteries of essential oils to crafting your blends, and from discovering their diverse applications to incorporating them seamlessly into your daily life, you've embarked on a transformative journey toward well-being and balance.

In the essence of our exploration, remember that the magic of essential oils lies not only in their potent scents but also in the mindful and safe practices that accompany their use. Dilute, experiment, and find your unique blend that resonates with your senses and elevates your life.

Whether you've delved into the world of DIY blends for relaxation, found solace in pain-relieving elixirs, or harnessed the power of aromatherapy for focus and concentration, you now possess a treasure trove of knowledge to enrich your daily life.

As you navigate the vast landscape of essential oils, always keep the title of our journey in mind: "How to Use Essential Oils for Beginners: A Step-By-Step Guide to DIY Aromatherapy Recipes for Anxiety Relief, Sleep

Remedies, All-Natural Cleaning Products, Skin Care, Pain Management, and More." Let it be your compass, guiding you through moments of tranquility, supporting your well-being, and enhancing the tapestry of your daily experiences.

May your days be fragrant, your nights restful, and your spirit uplifted by the aromatic wonders you've embraced. Until our scents intertwine again, keep exploring, experimenting, and savoring the delightful world of essential oils.

With aromatic regards.

www.ingramcontent.com/pod-product-compliance
Lightning Source LLC
Chambersburg PA
CBHW061006260726
48661CB00005B/2075